"Only you can help yourself…"

-Ancient Proverb

Table of Contents

This book is dedicated to my father, Ray Lawry, who always reminded me that the biggest room in the world was the room for improvement.

Why nobody is overweight

For many years I was frustrated with the terms *overweight, underweight and obesity,* as they were descriptions used by an outdated system called the Body Mass Index (BMI). This system is the model of choice for many medical and private weight loss programs and clinics. It determines your height and weight and then plots these numbers on a graph that categorizes you as being underweight, normal, or overweight.

I knew it did not describe accurately what was changing *inside* your body, because after I gained 20 pounds of muscle in 2001, I was categorized as being overweight, even though my body fat percentage did not change and remained a healthy 15%.

To understand the BMI system and to see why it is still in use today, despite its inaccuracies, we will have to go back over 200 years to an explanation given by a man in Belgium.

A Brief History of the BMI

The first known country to begin measuring people for obesity was Belgium in the late 19th century. They hired a mathematician named Lambert Adolph Quetelet, to devise a quick and simple formula to measure large numbers of people for the purpose of allocating health funding. The project had nothing to do with weight control, but he wanted to find out if height had anything to do with what could be determined as *normal* weight.

He discovered that weight varied not in proportion to height, but in proportion to the square of the height of most people. In 1832 he came up with the Quetelet Index of Obesity, which measured levels of obesity by dividing a person's weight (in kilograms) by the square of his or her height (in inches).

The formula was w/h2.

For the next 100 years it was not used or written about and began to vanish from the literature. In the late 1940's, medical insurance groups began again to use variables of height and weight for determining health risks, such as cardiovascular risk, associated with having too much *weight*. For many years doctors could not agree on which height or weight combination put a person at risk and they had no single number or system that would make it easy for them to promote.

In 1972, obesity researcher, Ancel Keyes, published *"Indices of Relative Weight and Obesity"*, which summarized his study of over 7400 men, from five different countries. He concluded that the best group predictor of a normal fat percentage was, in his opinion, the Quetlet formula. Keyes renamed this formula the Body Mass Index (BMI) and defined thresholds that would determine a normal weight situation.

Boring...

At first, the thresholds were established at the 85th percentile of BMI for each sex: 27.8% for men and 27.3% for women. It became an international standard for the measuring of obesity in 1980, and was introduced to the public in the late 1990's by the World Health Organization (WHO). The WHO is a group of health professionals put together by the United Nations to promote various agendas on behalf of their member group. In 1988, the first Canadian guidelines for describing a healthy weight were first introduced. They were based on the BMI system.

In 1998, The National Institute of Health (NIH), begins to promote the BMI to doctors and wants them to warn patients of the dangers of being too *heavy*.

Hang on…we're almost there.

In late 1998 the NIH changed the thresholds and consolidated the top end of "normal" for all adults, even though the relationship between body fat is *different* for each sex. The new cutoffs for both sexes were now 25 for normal and 30 for obese. They also included a new category called *overweight*, which included everyone who was just over *normal* but not quite *obese*. The WHO also endorsed this new protocol.

Overnight it was estimated that 35 million people in North America become overweight or obese without doing anything; they were just sleeping!

An updated version, dated April 11th, 2011, provides 6 different categories for people taking the BMI. It will now determine you as being:

1)   Underweight
2)   Normal (healthy)
3)   Overweight
4)   Obese Class 1
5)   Obese Class 2
6)   Obese Class 3

The medical/insurance business now has numbers to use, and an easy inexpensive way to diagnose a weight condition. All you need is a scale and a tape measure. And they also have a new health condition to target and treat...

You guessed it – 'overweight'.

In his original paper, Keyes warned against using the BMI for individual diagnosis, as it does not take into consideration individual variables such as fat percentages, muscle mass, bone structure, age or sex. Also, there is no physiological or scientific reason to square a person's height. Quetelet had to square the height to get a formula that matched the overall data that he had collected. In other words, if you can't fix the data, you need to rig the formula.

Have we Changed Much?

The punch line is we are still using this ancient system today. The BMI has hardly changed in 30 years and is still maintained in our health system and still promoted by medical groups such as the WHO, Health Canada, and in my province, The British Columbia Medical Association. It is also promoted as it keeps the public uninformed of any other options, keeps profits up for the medical/insurance business, and promotes more visits to the doctor's office for consultations and possible prescriptions of their "weight loss" drug of choice - *Orlistat*. This drug is a fat blocker and has some nasty side effects.

The BMI is still promoted by all of the major UN countries including Canada, and it is very unfortunate to see on Health Canada's website the citing following information:

> *"...The BMI (weight(kg) height(m)2 is not a direct measure of body fat, but is the most useful indicator to date of health risks associated with under and overweight. However, it should be considered a rough guide because it may not correspond to the same degree of fatness in different individuals..."*

Due to the incorrect science of the BMI, you can see why nobody is overweight. In fact, it is actually a misdiagnosis of any weight or health related condition. Any illness, injury or death caused by medical procedures, prescriptions or related causes is called *Iatrogenesis*. It was the third leading cause of death in North America in 2004 and is now rapidly becoming number one.

Please be aware of this situation the next time you or a loved one are given any advice, procedures or pills from those connected to the medical business.

If you find this confusing and contradictory, you are not alone. I find it embarrassing that this is what our nation's Health Care system is promoting as weight management. So, I felt compelled to offer a new model based on science, logic, and common sense.

A new model for weight control

My new model is based on the science of body composition, which can accurately determine what a normal or healthy weight is for you. Body composition is the sum total of the three main types of weight that can change in the body due to a variety of lifestyle factors. Theses weights are bone, muscle and fat. Since all other types of weight do not change significantly over time, measuring one's composition gives the best indication of what *type* of weight is changing in your body. It provides the necessary information to target the specific type(s) of weight that you may need to *gain* or *lose*.

For many years I was using skin fold calipers which are a widely accepted way to determine the fat percentage component of a person's body composition. I needed more information because we know that there are three weight components required to accurately measure body composition, which is the combined weights of fat, muscle, and bone. I began researching and trying new DEXA X-ray techniques that could also measure bone density. This added one more component to my testing package and it was proving to be both successful and acceptable to my clients. I was still a little frustrated, though, as I did not have an accurate or reliable way of measuring changes in muscle weight. I was using a hand grip device that only gave an overall value of your muscle strength, and as muscle can change fairly quickly in some individuals, I wanted to track those changes more effectively.

In 2004 my radiologist called me and said he had just acquired new software that could measure all three components of body composition and asked me if I would like to be scanned as his first guinea pig. I was elated and booked in right away, anticipating that this was the key diagnostic tool for developing a comprehensive new model. The software measures your *total* body composition and produces a print out of your scores.

Here were my scan numbers:

- Bone Density (T-score)   4.1
- Lean Muscle   48kg
- Fat   14.5%

The results showed that I was in a healthy range for all three weights which meant what I weighed on the bathroom scales was irrelevant. It shows that I had a healthy weight regardless of what my total weight was. My total weight was 208lbs, which is neither good nor bad - it was just the total of *all* my weights at that time.

What happened next accelerated my quest for developing a new model for weight control. In late 2004, one of my clients came to me in a state of confusion, complaining that his insurance company was going to charge him an extra $3000 for being *overweight.*

He was especially confused since he had recently passed a required fitness and medical examination which included a body fat measurement test. His body fat measured 22% which is within healthy ranges for males of his age. Testing also revealed that he had large muscles and dense bones.

So why was he being charged extra for being *overweight?* I told Kevin (my client) that according to the Life Insurance System, his heavy muscles and bone put him over their "recommended" weight range. I explained how many companies use the BMI system. I said it would measure your height and weight but cannot accurately measure body composition, which is the new way to determine what a healthy weight is for an individual. I told Kevin that BMI only looks at your height and weight and does not take into consideration weights that can change often such as muscle or fat.

For example, **only extra fat weight** can put you out of a healthy range, as muscle and bone are healthy necessary tissues *no matter how much you have*. Kevin was in an acceptable body composition range even though he was 5'9" and weighed 219 lbs. Kevin's tone became more agitated as he replied, "Do you mean that I'm *not* overweight?"

"That's right," I replied. "There is actually no such weight condition."

I told Kevin that I would call the Director of the Insurance Company, explain to him the principles of body composition, and hopefully make Kevin exempt from an extra payment.

Kevin didn't believe me.

I arranged a meeting the next week and told the Director that Kevin was actually being penalized for having lots of healthy, heavy, muscle and bone. I explained that *all* of his weights were in healthy ranges and that there was no valid reason for him to be called "overweight". In fact, I asked him what part of Kevin was "overweight", for which he had no answer! It turned out that the company accepted my explanations about body composition and offered Kevin a normal rate for his policy. The whole experience prompted me to create a new model for weight management which offers new technology, logical weight explanations, and natural solutions for adjusting your body composition.

Prior to DEXA scans there had been no general consensus as to what actually determined a healthy or normal weight for individuals. This is now changing as more fitness and health professionals are endorsing the Body Composition scan for determining weight control strategies. The old definition of a healthy weight was based on the outdated BMI model, which cannot measure individual changes in body composition. Muscle, bone and fat, can change inside your body and the BMI cannot measure these important differences.

Here is the new definition:

> *A healthy weight is achieved when your body composition (fat, muscle and bone) is within recommended ranges.*

To measure and determine if your body composition is in recommended ranges, you will need to take a DEXA body composition scan, DEXA stands for Dual Emission X-ray Absorptiometry. This system accurately measures your weights and is the new gold standard for measuring body composition in the world.

This may come as a surprise, but knowing these internal weights is far more important than knowing the number on your bathroom scale.

You may need or want to lose some fat weight, gain a little muscle, or build up valuable bone density to reach a healthy weight, and I will explain later how this can be accomplished.

DEXA is a low radiation X-ray scan that accurately measures your levels of fat, muscle and bone - *the only weights that change when you gain or lose weight.* This is important because you need to know what *kind* of weight is changing inside your body over time, especially if you are concerned about bone loss.

It is also important to know that this model is not about "weight loss", which is a term that is often used to market a program or service. Any program that uses these words really cannot tell you what kind of weight you will be losing and this is *not* a healthy situation. It has been my experience that those marketing this concept do not understand the real issues of weight control and offer only false or misleading information.

All the information and suggestions provided in this book have proven to be effective for dozens of clients over the past five years. This book offers over twenty different strategies for adjusting fat, muscle, or bone to help you reach your recommended levels. It offers challenging new information to achieve these goals, and explains all the reasons why there are no such conditions as *"overweight"*, *"underweight"*, *"obese"*, or *"ideal weight"*.

This book is your guide to my new model and it's designed to help you *lose* or *gain* the kind of weight that is best suited for **you**.

The model is based on the principles of body composition, and the program I teach is called The Healthy Weight® Program. To reap the most benefits, take your time and really commit to each chapter of this book, as it may take up to 12 months to see positive results.

Thank you for your interest in developing and maintaining a healthy weight, and I wish you all the best in your efforts. I say this with all sincerity and honesty; you may now throw out your bathroom scale.

Let me tell you why.

Body composition is more important than your *weight*

We've all stepped off the bathroom scales and said "Crap, I've just gained a few pounds..." or, "Wow, how did I *lose* all this weight?"

Chances are you have experienced both scenarios, but did you ever wonder what *kind* of weight was lost or gained? Standing on the bathroom scale or any other kind of scale will not give you that information as they can only measure your *total body weight*, and not the internal weights which may change over time. To understand this concept fully, it's important to know that there are five main types of weight in the human body. They are:

- Fat
- Muscle
- Bone
- Organs
- Fluids

Two of these weights, fluids and organs, do not change significantly over time and do not need to be measured. The other three can and *do* change throughout our lives. A sudden increase or loss of fat weight is the most common scenario.

Muscle loss or gain is the next most common, with bone loss or gain being the least common. Since these weights can change throughout our lives I have termed them *active weights*. There are recommended ranges for each active weight and it is important to monitor them on a regular basis to see which ones need to be adjusted to maintain a healthy weight. Outlined below are the most common reasons why your active weights have shifted over time:

- If you are inactive, you can gain fat and lose muscle
- If you start a fitness program, especially one that involves resistance training, you can gain muscle, increase bone mass, and lose fat
- When you begin and continue a low caloric or starvation type diet, you can lose muscle and gain fat

- You can lose fat with a dedicated program of diet, exercise and lifestyle management
- Muscle is often lost as we age (called *sarcopenia*)
- Bone loss can happen if you are inactive, hormonally unbalanced, or do not eat the essential foods to maintain good bone density
- Bone gains can be made with a dedicated diet, exercise and lifestyle program
- Toxic internal weight can be gained over a long period of time. It also can be lost with a supervised program of detoxification

Here's a very common scenario:

> Over a period of time you could gain fifteen pounds of fat, especially if you have become sedentary. During that same period you could have lost fifteen pounds of muscle. Standing on your bathroom scale things still look the same, but you notice some changes. You may notice you are loosening that darned belt a few notches too...

In this scenario two of your active weights, fat and muscle, have shifted over time within your body. In order to accurately measure which weight and how much of that weight has shifted, we'll need to go *inside* your body for the answers.

To do this, I use the safe, low emission DEXA X-ray scan. The scan takes about 20 minutes. A scanning apparatus passes over your body while you lay flat on your back. As it scans it generates a signature of your body composition. Upon completion, it generates a picture of the results in three specific categories:

1) Bone density
2) Lean tissue (muscle)
3) Body fat percentage

Body fat is recorded as a percentage of your total weight and can be converted to either pounds or kilograms for fat loss strategies. Muscle is recorded as part of your *total* lean tissue score which is everything in your body minus bone and fat (including organs too). It is measured in grams and although it measures all tissue, only *muscle* changes significantly. So, we take two tests, and subtract your initial score from your second score. The difference is the change in your muscle weight over time. Ideally, we hope it goes up!

Bone weight is recorded as a density and is referred to as your Bone Mass Density, or BMD. Your density score is also compared to an international system known as the *T Score*. The *T Score* is a numbering system which rates the density of bone. I only use DEXA for recording changes, as it is not that accurate for diagnosing weak or "porous" bones, more commonly known as "osteoporosis". I will talk more about that in Chapter 6.

The Outdated BMI Model

Body mass Index (BMI) is the model of weight diagnosis which is promoted by the medical community in most countries. The main problem with this model is that it is not accurate in measuring weights that can change in your body such as muscle and fat. Another problem is that if you "buy" into this diagnostic system, there is a possibility that you will also be subject to their three different "treatment" plans, which may be inappropriate for your situation. Here are the three scenarios, as outlined in the British Columbia Medical Association's (BCMA) "Guidelines for Physicians."

1)   If you are diagnosed as being "overweight" or "obese" you may be recommended to follow *lifestyle management* course of action which basically states "*refer the patient to a weight loss program*"

2)   Pharmacological management is next.   This guide states it may be necessary "*only after dietary, exercise and behavioral approaches have failed*". The guidelines then go on to say "*...currently Orlistat (brand name Xenical®), is the only medication marketed for the long term treatment of obesity, available in Canada.*"

Orilast is fat blocker and its side effects are nasty. They include fecal incontinence, oily leaks, diarrhea, abdominal bloating, flatulence, vomiting and limited *weight loss* results. The guide continues to go on...

3)   **Surgical   Intervention   (bariatric)   is   also available   and,   *"...gastric   bypass   and laparoscopic band surgery are the most common forms of surgery procedures"***

The BMI scale was based on the Insurance driven model that was first conceived in the 1940's. Companies back then needed a quick and easy way to determine if a client had a risk factor for Cardiovascular Disease (CVD) and doctors were convinced that height/weight charts were good *risk* indicators. The more risk factors that the insurers could find, the higher you paid for your insurance. It was and still is a profitable business that often has inadequate health assessments for determining your risk factors.

The medical insurance business has made money over the past 70 years using a system that is obsolete, inaccurate and in many cases blatantly incorrect in their diagnosis for weight and risk factors. They also may use a kind of fear based tactic to help you buy into their program. I recommend avoiding any person or program that says you should lose weight or go on a weight loss plan. It is incorrect information. This shows a lack of knowledge of body composition, and a lack of respect for your individual needs.

I have tested dozens of people who were deemed overweight and obese, who had perfectly normal body compositions, and were very pleased to know how their composition determined the best course of action.

So if you feel that the medical insurance model is not one that will benefit you with your body composition issues, and you are looking for an alternative, I would like to offer you the concepts of the *Healthy Weight Program*. This program interprets your personal DEXA X-ray data (fat, muscle and bone) and provides natural solutions for adjusting them into healthy ranges.

Since the introduction of the body composition software for DEXA scanners in 2004, all other weight measuring systems have become obsolete, along with any suggested weight ranges which they may offer. The following systems are no longer used in my new model of weight control:

- Height/weight charts
- Body Mass Index (BMI) formulas
- Bioimpedance scales
- Body fat calipers
- Girth measurements (hip to waist ratios)
- Weight scales
- Underwater weighing

We also do not use any of the following terms which are associated with these systems such as:

- Overweight
- Underweight
- Obese or obesity
- Ideal weight
- Recommended weight
- Weight loss

It is important at this point to know that there is a completely new way to measure and define your overall weight situation using new technology and terminology.

Are you ready for your first scan?

Contact me using the navigation at the end of this book and we can provide you with information on all of the available DEXA clinics in British Columbia, Canada. These clinics are also aware of my new model and The *Healthy Weight Program*. This book can be read without taking a scan, but I do recommend you have one as soon as possible, as the next steps will have more personal meaning.

If you are outside of B.C., contact Radiology Clinics in your area that offer the body composition protocol and proceed with a scan. Contact me after your scan and we can provide you with an on-line/telephone coaching service for your benefit.

What is your healthy weight?

With the aid of DEXA scans, current fitness and health guidelines, I have developed a new definition of a healthy weight.   Here it is again:

> *A healthy weight is achieved when your body composition (fat, muscle and bone) is within recommended ranges.*

This new definition is based on your own personal body composition results. For example:

Let's say your body composition is within healthy ranges and you weigh 180 lbs. This is your healthy *total* weight for you at this time, even if height/weight, BMI charts, or scales are suggesting otherwise.   If you gain a little bone or muscle, this will not affect your current status. You could gain 12 pounds of muscle or gain 4 pounds of bone and *still* be in a healthy range. If your muscle level was high to begin with, you could afford to lose a little of this kind of weight and still be in range. If you gain a little too much fat though, this could affect your status, as only fat can put you out of a healthy range - not muscle or bone.   Both are healthy weights and we need them for a healthy life.

I have recorded many people with heavy bones and muscles who thought they were 'overweight' according to the BMI charts, yet they had a perfectly healthy body composition.

Another example is the following scenario I had. A female client came to my program who had weighed 170 lbs. for over ten years, and during that time had been told by many people and fitness centers that she was *overweight*. She did not feel unhealthy or that she had a weight problem but soon became very self conscious of her size and weight. After taking a DEXA scan and discovering that she had a good body composition, she was very relieved, and became far more self confident about her body and self esteem.

I have also measured individuals who were *underweight* according to the BMI scale, who also had a healthy body composition. They were just small people with lower than average muscle or low body fat content. I have also measured individuals who were *obese* according to the BMI scale. These people, mostly big, heavily muscled men, who also had a healthy weight. They just were big in all the right areas from years of lifting heavy weights!

> What is often hard to grasp about this
> new model is that all of the old methods
> of measuring weight are no longer used.

I do not suggest weight amounts that you need to be or "should" be at this time. For example, I have overheard weight loss centre employees saying to a client, "You should weigh between 130 and 140 pounds." This is unfair and inaccurate as there is no scientific reason for saying this. What I have learned is that the majority of these centers are sales driven, not *results* driven.

There are three main composition categories that need to be adjusted or changed to reach a healthy weight. You may want or need to:

1) Increase your bone weight (density)
2) Increase your muscle weight (strength)
3) Lose excess fat weight (%)

You are given a fairly broad range for each active weight and it is up to you to decide which one(s) and what "weight" changes you want to make. These recommended ranges will be outlined in the next chapter. Please know that there is no such term as "weight loss" in my program. For example, you will **never** hear me say: *"You need to lose ten pounds, or, let's lose some weight!"*

I may say you could lose some fat, gain some bone or gain some more muscle, as these are the reasonable and truthful ways to express the new way I determine your individual situation.

I offer information designed to help you reach a recommended range for all three weights and assist you in reaching these goals by offering only natural non-drug based solutions. Let's find out what they are next.

The room for improvement

In the next sections, I will be sharing with you some of the most effective ways to adjust your active weights (fat & muscle) so that you can achieve a Healthy Weight. Before you start, it is important to prepare yourself for the real and often life changing results that can happen when your composition begins to shift into healthier ranges.

Once you have taken the DEXA body comp scan, you may want to make some changes or improvements. Real change can happen with some basic strategies, and one of the best ways to start is by writing down your *intents, goals and action steps*.

Your intents describe how you want to feel and what state of being you desire for the long term.

Intents Example:

> "I intend to feel positive about all the changes I will be making, and look forward to enjoying long term health benefits."

Now write down your goals. Goals need to be reasonable, attainable, and measurable over time. They provide a baseline for change and improvement.

Goals Example:

> "I want to lose 12% body fat, which I feel is attainable in the next 9-12 months."

Now write down the Action Steps. These are things that you can do right away to begin the process of achieving your intents and goals.

Action Steps Example:

> "I'm going to buy a new pair of running shoes, hire a trainer, and set aside three hours a week for exercise."

Prepare for Change

1)   If you desire to change your composition, especially fat weight; make changes because you want and feel you *deserve* the change.

Avoid being influenced by anyone or any marketing which says you *should* be a certain weight, size or shape.

2)   Visualize your new self and see yourself as you *really* want to be. Repeat to yourself the reasons for deserving a healthy weight. Practice these on a daily basis to reinforce your vision and help your body *know* that change is coming. This "rehearsal" of how you *want* to be can prepare you for what you *will* be in the near future.

3)   Set aside time for yourself. Take time off to do the things you love to do or haven't done for a long time. This is not selfish - it is wise to invest in yourself first.

4)   Learn and practice the skills of becoming more assertive. This style of behavior means that you always work on being balanced, healthy, positive, pro-active, helpful, and compassionate. It means that you work to create win/win situations and value principles such as honesty, integrity and courage. The overall feeling that you have when you become more assertive is this; *everyone in my world counts and so do I, but I count first!* This behavior will help you become more successful in meeting your body composition goals and sustaining them for a lifetime.

5)   Create a support team to assist you in handling the tough times and those days when you feel like going back to old ways which could sabotage your new efforts.

6)   Weight control is not always about "losing weight," it is about gaining new information, skills and confidence to keep your body in a healthy balance. Rather than avoiding food, you need to feed yourself high quality, nutrient dense, whole, natural foods that are full of micronutrients for optimal health. Prepare to eat 4-7 meals per day of nourishing foods that keep your bones, muscles and fat levels in healthy ranges. When you give the body what it needs, it no longer needs to store fat, waiting for you to feed it what it really needs. Fat loss becomes more attainable and sustainable over a longer period of time.

It is also important that you prepare for how people will perceive your changes. It is often hard for people to accept change in others, as they may see you only as they wish, not as *you* can truly be in a new body, shape or size. It is not important how *they* think or feel about your changes, it is only important what *you* think and feel about your changes.

Prepare to look, feel, move, and even sound differently. Changing your body composition can affect all of these areas more than you may have suspected. These changes are positive and you need to know that it is natural and healthy to have a recommended body composition. Let's look inside your body and see what can change next.

Your recommended weight ranges

I could start with fat but I prefer to start with bone weight due to the important role it plays in our body. Failing to recognize bone loss at a young or middle age could lead to fragile or brittle bones later on in your life. Bone loss can often be more detrimental than having too much fat.

1) Bone Weight

The DEXA scan passes over your body and records bone as a density measurement called the *Adult T Score*.

> The minimum recommended T Score for both males and females is zero (0).

If your score is between 0 and -1.4, there may be indication of initial bone loss. This kind of bone loss is termed *Osteopenia*. If your score is between -1.4 and -2.4, then there is indication of a term called *Osteoporosis*. Scores below -2.4 indicate more severe bone loss where the bone is actually becoming porous, and hence the name *Osteoporosis*, which means *porous bone*.

The International Society for Clinical Densitometry (ISCD) suggests that any score above zero is considered normal and healthy for adults. I feel that the higher your score is, the better it is for you. It helps you to have more strength for activities and sports and also helps prevent bone loss for the future.

We have recorded female scores as high as 2.8, which is not uncommon for athletic folks. I was surprised when my own scan recorded a score of 4.1 which is very high for males. The radiologist who was interpreting my scan was shocked and told me that I was *very* dense. All I could think of to say was, *"Thanks?!"*

In this Chapter 7, I will show you how to get your bone density as high as possible.

2) Muscle Weight

The DEXA software measures all of the body's lean tissue and records it in grams. Your total Lean Tissue score in grams represents all lean tissue including those such as your lungs, kidneys, spleen and muscles. Since muscles are your only tissue which changes on a regular basis, any changes in the Lean G score indicates changes in muscle weight only.

For example:

> If your initial score was 45,000g and your second score was 45,500g you have gained 500 grams (0.5kg) of muscle between scans. Conversely, if your score goes down on the second scan to 44,500g you have *lost* 500 grams of muscle. This can unfortunately happen, especially if you attempt to "starve" yourself by trying various low caloric diets. This will be explained fully in Chapter 8.

Muscle weight can also be gained quite rapidly as well, especially if you follow a progressive weight training program. Men will show more gain than women on this kind of a program, but it is important to remember that having strong heavy muscles does not mean you are *overweight*. It only means that you have good healthy tissue for sports and activity!

There are no current recommended ranges for Lean (G) Tissue, but we offer a general range based on minimal muscular requirements and our experience with hundreds of DEXA scans:

Females, greater than **32,000 Lean grams** (32kg)
Males, greater than **42,000 Lean grams** (42kg)

You may also take the Canadian Standard test for muscle strength and endurance. To reach a recommended score you need to be in the *Average, Above Average*, or the *Good* category. Measuring your bone and muscle on a regular basis is a valuable health screening practice for one main reason: you do not want to be *losing* these two important weights.

3) Fat Weight

The DEXA scan scores body fat as a percentage of your total body weight.

For example:

Let's say you are a 200 lbs. man and you have a fat percentage score of 20%.

This means you have 40 lbs. of fat on your body. This may seem like a lot of fat, but actually it is within the healthy ranges for a man. We have measured some males who have as little as 7%, but it is not recommended to drop below 5%, due to the hormonal needs of fat for testosterone production.

It is important that females do not drop below 13%. Low energy and hormonal imbalances are two of the most common symptoms. The loss of menses is also an unhealthy result of a low body fat percentage.

Recommended Body Fat Percentage ranges:

For Males less than 40 years old: **8-22 %**
  Greater than 40 years old: **12-24 %**

For Females less than 40 years old: **16-33 %**
  Greater than 40 years old: **18-36 %**

Fat weight can change quite often due to various factors, so it is important to monitor its changes on a regular basis. If your fat percentage is above the recommended levels, you may be a little *over-fat* but this does not mean that you are *overweight*. Just a reminder - there is no such condition! If you are a little over the suggested ranges for fat at this time, you can change it into a healthy range with some dedicated effort on your part and some of our suggestions listed in Chapter 9.

4) Toxic Weight

Did you know that over time you can gain up to five pounds or more from toxic waste matter in your body? It sounds a little gross, but we are all subject to environmental toxins, food additives, preservatives, chemicals, poor dietary choices and a lack of exercise. Some or all of these factors can contribute to a build up of toxic matter in the body. These toxins often end up in the colon, liver, kidneys and the lymphatic system.

There are no recommended amounts for toxic weight loss as everyone will have different levels to begin with. We can however recommend some kind of detoxification program prior to starting any health program.

Here are some examples of detoxification:

- Colonic Irrigation
- Ionic Detox Footbaths*
- Herbal Detox Programs
- FAR Infrared saunas

We have seen quite a lot of toxic weight loss due to these programs, and this is considered a good type of loss because it usually is unnecessary weight.

> I currently have one of the most advanced systems of removing toxic waste available. Call me for more information.

Did you know?

> We have recorded eight pounds of toxic loss due to a condition known as a *compacted colon.*   Toxic weight loss is a   natural   and   often   necessary procedure, as the body often needs a spring cleaning.   Note, all toxic weight loss programs should be done with the aid of a qualified practitioner.

Your Personal Healthy Weight

Now that you have the target ranges for all of the active weights, you can see where you are doing well and see which areas which need may attention.   You may want or need to lose some fat weight, gain a little muscle, or build back some valuable bone density.

> When all of these weights are in their recommended ranges you have reached

a personal <u>healthy weight</u>, one that is right for you and you only!

Two examples of a Healthy Weight:

1)   Female, 56 years old:

Bone Density (T- score):   1.5
Lean Tissue: 36,656g
Body Fat: 34%

2)   Male, 42 years old:

Bone Density (T-score):   2.6
Lean Tissue: 42,456g
Body Fat: 18%

The man in this example could weigh between 180 to 220 lbs. and the woman 120 to 145 lbs. and it would make no difference, as they are both in healthy ranges. These are two examples of how I now measure and determine a *Healthy Weight*. It is only based on the new DEXA body composition assessment and not from the numbers you see on your bathroom scale, or from numbers you may see on height/weight or BMI charts! For twenty years I used skin fold calipers for measuring body fat, which is still acceptable for some situations, but I have no longer used them since starting DEXA in 2005.

The main concept of this chapter is to realize there is a new way to measure and monitor your weight. You no longer need to be influenced by the scales or by people trying to convince you how much you *should or should not weigh,* based on their opinion or that of a particular measuring system.   You no longer need to be influenced by the latest *diet* or *weight loss* program or those who are attempting to sell you something that use the terms *diet* or *weight loss* in their marketing material.

The people promoting these services or products know little about what kind of weight you will be losing and have no idea how to monitor changes even if you are successful at losing "weight." Most "weight loss clinics" that I have seen are only concerned about selling you a program, and not about improving your body composition, well-being, or health.

We now have the technology and knowledge to truly understand what determines a natural healthy weight. This knowledge is powerful and will be valuable in helping you to achieve and maintain a healthy weight throughout your life.

Next step – *are you ready for achieving a Healthy Weight?*

Creating healthy bones

Have you ever wondered *how* your bones can become brittle or break and *why* this increases with age? To better understand how bone is gained and lost, we first need to offer a short introduction on bone:

- The human body contains 208 bones which make up approximately 30% of your total weight
- Bones assist in the production of blood cells and provide a valuable storage area for minerals
- Bone is active living tissue that is primarily collagen fibers reinforced by calcium and other minerals

- It is in a constant state of turnover as various hormonal actions work together to create more bone and keep it strong
- Our bones are alive and contain channels which blood flows through. Cells called *osteoclast*s travel among these channels constantly looking for, and removing old bone
- While doing so they often create small 'holes'
- Cells called *Osteoblasts* then arrive on the scene with calcium and minerals to fill in these holes and create new bone

The process mentioned above is an ongoing one called *bone remodeling*. When we are younger this process repeats itself every three to four months, but slows down with age. Bone loss occurs when this process of making new bone falls behind the process of removing old bone.

Initial bone loss is termed Osteopenia as we mentioned earlier, and more severe loss is termed Osteoporosis (porous bone). Both bone conditions are actually *symptoms* of a more complex metabolic problem which creates porous and/or weakened bones. The root causes of porous bone and bone loss are mainly due to *bone remodeling dysfunction (BRD), which is a new description that replaces "osteoporosis"*. BRD occurs when osteoclasts and osteoblasts begin to slow down due to a combination of factors. These factors include:

1)   **Poor dietary choices.** This usually means that there is not enough calcium and mineral rich foods in the diet.

2)   **Lack of exercise.** Exercise stimulates osteoblasts to form new bone and moderate exercise has been shown to increase bone density.

3)   **Hormonal Imbalances.** Low testosterone in both males and females is linked to bone loss. Elevated estrogen and lowered progesterone levels in females can also contribute to bone loss. An unbalanced parathyroid gland can also weaken bone. It is responsible for regulating calcium in the body and needs to be functioning well to maintain its role in bone strength.

4)   **Poor calcium absorption.** Most calcium can only be absorbed in the small intestine, where it requires ideal pH conditions. It is often excreted or put back into the tissues, joints and blood where it can build up to toxic levels.

5)   **Acidosis.** An acidic body will often require alkalizing minerals to counter the negative effects of too much acid. For the body to achieve this condition, calcium (a dominant alkalizing mineral) can be drawn out of the bones to assist in this process, which contributes to bone loss.

6)   **Low stomach acid.** If your levels are low, overall digestion and absorption (including calcium and minerals) can be affected.

7)   **Osteoclasts and osteoblasts slowing down**. There are three scenarios in which this condition may happen:

   i)   **Over consumption of dairy products**. Research and DEXA scans are showing that countries with the highest consumption of cow based dairy products also suffer from the highest incidence of BRD. Milk is not digested or processed well in the human as only about 30% is absorbed. This leads to lower absorption rates, and Osteoblast slowdown. It is also acidic and can lead to increased acidosis.

   ii)   **Over consumption of calcium with low bio-availability**. These include calcium derived from rocks, shells, coral and other sources that are often sold in supplements.

   iii) **Bisphosphonate Drugs**. There are currently three kinds that are approved for use in Canada. They are Alendronate (Fosamax), Etidronate (Didrocal), and Risedronate (Actonel).

Both situations *i* and *ii* cause the Osteoblasts to process a lot of calcium which causes them to become exhausted and slow down their abilities to create new bone.

Here's an analogy:

> If you exercised once a day you would probably be able to handle the stress of it, but if you tried to work out three or four times a day, you would become exhausted and probably quit.

The same is true for osteoblasts. They can handle only so much stress from processing calcium. Overloading their abilities can cause them to slow down considerably, which in turn slows down the remodeling process and results in further bone loss. The human body prefers natural, organic, and *very* bio-available sources of calcium and usually in smaller doses that are currently being recommended.

Client Example:

> A female client in 2008 increased her bone density from -0.1 to a positive 0.9 in one year by eating more alkalizing foods and those containing organic calcium and minerals.

Beware of Bisphosphonate drugs which are prescribed to increase bone density. The initial results of this drug therapy look good, as often the bone density will go up after one year. The problem is that this bone is old, dry, brittle and not new strong bone matrix. Drug companies use these first year results only and make them sound like their product is helping when actually these drugs contribute to weaker bones.

Here's what really happens.

These drugs slow down or destroy the 'old bone' removing abilities of the osteoclasts. This causes the old brittle bone to build up which eventually begins to weaken and crumble! Osteoblasts (*hole fillers*) have fewer holes to fill, less work to perform, and their abilities begin to deteriorate when osteoclasts (*hole makers*) are not functioning. The process accelerates after two to three years, and bone loss after five years can lead to fractures of the femur and other large bones. For the past seven years, my experience with the effects of various "bone density increasing" drugs has proven to be disastrous. We have records of clients whose bone loss was due to the action of drugs that were prescribed to *prevent* bone loss!

Client Example:

> A new 56 year old female client had an initial T score of -2.2, which is quite low. She was prescribed Alendronate (brand name: Fosamax) and went for a second scan one year later. Her score had dropped to -2.9. A third scan after three years revealed a score of - 3.1! Her physician had tried two different drugs

and changed the dosage three times in an unsuccessful attempt to stop her bone loss.

It is unfortunate that these drugs are being prescribed to *treat* a symptom called Osteoporosis in Canada and the United States. The term has now been raised to the status of a "disease", in much of the newest medical literature, which I believe is a misguided description.

The condition is actually a short term **healing** *mechanism that did not receive enough assistance from its owner and has turned into a longer term health problem. The body, in its wisdom, will take calcium and minerals from the bones and deliver it to an area that requires it as a high priority. The bones are storehouses for minerals and the body will draw on these reserves in times of need, or when it is out of balance. The bones must be replenished otherwise unhealthy, weak or porous bones become the consequence.*

It is challenging to realize that *modern medicine* has not yet discovered the root causes of porous or weakened bone and the natural ways to stop and reverse it. As mentioned, *Osteoporosis* is just a word that describes the long term consequences of a short term healing process. The medical establishment promotes the word, but offers little for natural ways to treat the root causes. The first line treatment they are recommending is bisphosphonates.

There are currently a number of lawsuits in motion against the companies that produce these drugs, especially Fosamax, as it has been linked to *Osteonecrosis*. This is Osteoporosis of the jaw, also known as "dead jaw". Merck, the company selling the drug Fosamax, *set aside over 40 million dollars* years ago evidently to fight these lawsuits.

Maybe they knew something we didn't...

> For more information on this subject, please refer to my new book coming up titled *"Osteoporosis - Disease or Healer?"*

Building Up Our Bones

Porous, thin or weakened bones can be prevented and reversed. Here are some new, natural and effective bone building strategies:

1)   Attempt to eat more absorbable forms of calcium and minerals, preferably in the form of raw food. The following foods contain calcium, magnesium, boron, copper, iodine, silicone, manganese, zinc, and chromium which are all good for bone health:

- Spirulina/algae
- Spinach

- Broccoli
- Kale
- Nettles
- Green leafy vegetables
- Sea vegetables (dulse etc.)
- Hazelnuts, brazil nuts
- Figs

2)   **Maintain an alkalizing diet** for good pH balance.

If your body becomes too acidic, a condition known as *acidosis* can occur. Calcium, a potent alkalizer, can be drawn out of the bones to "buffer" excess acid, and this contributes to bone loss. The human body prefers to be in a slightly *alkaline* state. This means we must provide it with good alkalizing foods to keep it in a state of balance.

The ideal pH of the blood is 7.365 and can be measured using new blood tests. A good alternative method is testing your saliva or urine with pH paper. For over 20 years I have been promoting the concepts of pH balancing, and now there is a tremendous amount of literature to support the benefits of providing your body with the right ingredients to create an acid/alkaline balance. Research has shown that normal pH levels for most tissues and fluids in our bodies are alkaline. Here is a condensed version of what we have learned:

1)   The human body functions in its optimum state when it has lots of alkalizing foods and water to keep all bodily fluids in a state of balance known as *homeostasis*. This state helps the body to have more energy, lowers the incidence of headaches, joint stiffness and pain. It is also very helpful in preventing bone loss and in treating the root causes of Cellular Dysfunction (ie, *cancer*).

2)   The body has a tendency to become more acidic due to metabolic actions such as breathing, (carbonic acid) and exercising, (lactic acid) and it needs a constant supply of alkalizing foods and water to maintain *homeostasis*.

3)   From a food perspective, this means there needs to be approximately 70-80% alkalizing foods in your diet, and approximately 20-30% acidic foods. Here is a short list of common alkaline foods:

- Most fruits and veggies
- Uncooked or lightly steamed veggies are preferable such as: spinach, kale, celery, broccoli, carrots, fennel, and onions
- Green aquatic plants, such as algae & kelp
- Some nuts, such as almonds and walnuts
- Some grains such as spelt
- Alkalized water (pH of 7-10.5)

Here are common acid forming foods:

- Most meats (beef, ham, chicken & seafood)
- Most grains (read, rice & wheat products, etc.)
- Alcohol, soft drinks, coffee and non herbal teas
- All drugs
- Most dairy products, yogurts, & cheese
- Refined sugar, artificial ingredients & preservatives

4)   It is also important to lower your negative stress levels and your exposure to environmental, chemical or drug related toxins. They can have an impact on your ability to stay in a more alkaline state.

You can monitor your pH levels by purchasing pH litmus paper strips at health food stores, or talk to your local naturopath for specific ones to suit your needs. The full range of pH is measured on a scale between 0 - 14. Any reading above 7 is considered to be alkaline. Below 7 is considered to be more acidic. A reading of 7 is considered a neutral pH.

Most pH self-testing strips will display a range of pH from 5.6 (yellow in color) to 8.0 (blue in color). A neutral pH of 7 will display a dark green. To monitor your pH levels, take a strip of pH paper (one to two inches long) and pass it through a stream of urine, once in the morning, once in the afternoon and again in the evening. The same can be done with pH litmus paper using saliva, but urine is usually more accurate.

Ideally your paper will go from a light green color in the morning, to a darker green almost blue color in the afternoon, and then return to a green hue later at night.

The overall goal here is to get out of the yellow phase and into a greener state!

Being more alkalized can increase your mineral reserves, especially calcium and magnesium which are essential for many internal functions. Managing your pH levels and keeping them in healthy ranges is a powerful and beneficial way to maintain a *Healthy Weight*.

Back to our List

3)   **Start or maintain a moderate exercise program**. Examples are walking, hiking and resistance exercises such as weight training. They stimulate osteoblasts and can contribute to increased bone density and strength.

4)   **Increase Omega 3 "good oils" in your diet.** These essential oils help prevent calcium loss and contribute to lowering arterial inflammation. One of the main symptoms of arterial inflammation is elevated levels of total cholesterol and LDL, the so-called 'bad cholesterol'.

NOTE: Contrary to a lot of information you may have read or heard lately, high cholesterol is not a risk factor for "heart disease". It is actually a healer of the body and shows up in spades when the body's arteries are inflamed or damaged. It is only a <u>symptom</u> of a larger health problem called *intravascular stress*. Look for my next book coming all about it title *"Natural Solutions for a Healthy Heart"*. This book will shed more light on this controversial topic.

5)   **Maintain healthy *homocysteine* levels.** Elevated levels, especially in elderly people, have shown to contribute to bone loss.

6)   **Avoid soft drinks, corticosteroids & smoking.**

7)   **Start or maintain a negative stress reducing program.** Cortisol, the 'fight or flight' hormone is produced in the adrenal glands and can become elevated with negative stress. Elevated levels have a negative impact on bone remodeling.

8)   **Have your thyroid checked** on a regular basis for T3, T4 and TSH levels. Healthy

levels help to keep bone in top shape and prevent bone loss. It may be important to check for *parathyroid dysfunction*, especially if bone loss is sudden.   This gland is responsible for regulating calcium in the body and it can become overactive, causing *hyperparathyroidism* - a condition which leads to rapid bone loss.

I have recorded a *10 lbs. bone loss in one year* due to this condition. This is obviously not the kind of weight that you want to lose!

9)   **Monitor your levels of DHEA and Humane Growth Hormone (HGH)**. It is important to keep them as high as possible. Both can diminish as humans age and can be detrimental to bone health.

10)   **Increase your uptake of vitamin K and Vitamin D**.   Both are helpful in the formation of new bone. Sunshine is a natural and free source of vitamin D. Attempt to get 15-30 minutes a day before 11am and after 4pm, if possible.

Past Client Result:

By using a mixture of the above strategies I have recorded many increases in bone density. An increase of 23% over a fourteen month period has been our highest result to date. Not only is density increased with these techniques but the strength and integrity of the bone is enhanced as well.

This is challenging new information and I trust it may assist you towards a lifelong strategy for maintaining healthy bones.

Your *muscle* weight is next.

Maintain & improve healthy muscle weight

The human body has over 300 muscles that respond to our commands, propel us through the day, and give us a sense of strength and power.   Strong, healthy muscles are essential to have and to maintain throughout our life. To keep them in top shape it is up to us to provide them with adequate levels of resistance exercise on a regular basis.

Here are some examples:

- Jogging, fast walking, hiking, or biking
- Exercises which incorporate bodyweight (i.e. pushups, sit-ups, squats, etc.)
- Resistance bands (rubber tubes)
- Free weights or selective machine weight exercises

The results of your DEXA scan may show that you could gain a bit of muscle weight, and you may also want to gain some for your activities. I encourage a lifelong program of resistance training as it develops and maintains a good functional level of essential muscle. This will not cause you to become too bulky or "overweight", especially if you follow a gradual resistance program. If you want to make faster gains, there is a system known as *muscle pyramiding* which you can try.

Here's the basic technique of muscle pyramiding using a standard bicep curl as an example:

1)   Starting with a light weight (8lbs.), perform 12 repetitions
2)   Wait ten seconds, use a heavier weight, (10lbs.), and perform 7 reps
3)   Finish with a 12 lbs. weight and do 3 reps

Keep track of your workout weights and attempt this routine three or four times per week for three months.

4)   After three months, increase those weights with a small increment. Instead of starting with 8 lbs. move up to 10 lbs. then do your second set with 12 lbs. and finish up with 15 lbs.
5)   Attempt to increase these weights again after another one to two months and start with 15

lbs., take it to 20 lbs., then you should be able to finish with 25 lbs.

This technique can be used for all major muscles in the body and can be repeated at any time for further gains.

Remember, it is important that you be able to do the first 12 repetitions of any exercise confidently with ease.

If you cannot, you are stressing this muscle group. If this is the case, start your muscle building routine with a lower weight until 12 reps feels comfortable.

Client Result:

After a lengthy illness, Tony came to me wanting to gain back his fitness levels and especially his muscle size and strength. Using the pyramid method, he gained 22 lbs. of muscle in 12 months.

Keep in mind that men will develop more muscle weight than females due to naturally higher levels of testosterone, but females can also make some significant gains as well. A muscle weight gain of 6 lbs. is not unusual and can be very helpful for daily activities.

More tips for resistance training:

- Plan your workout when you have the most amount of energy in your day
- Perform a warm-up routine to facilitate blood flow and increase nerve stimulation
- Try different exercises and various apparatus for variety (i.e. Bosu balls, free weights, resistance bands or water workouts)
- Avoid the hype of synthetic steroids, growth hormones, and testosterone boosters to gain muscle weight. They can have adverse side effects and may harm your health in the long term.

Unfortunately, you can also *lose* muscle at certain times in your life, due to three metabolic problems called muscle atrophy, muscle sacrificing, and sarcopenia. *Take care to avoid these three scenarios as they will compromise your ability to maintain or gain more muscle.*

Muscle Atrophy

This situation usually arises from the old saying "if you don't use it you lose it". If you stop fitness activities, become sedentary or bedridden for any extended period, you can lose muscle size and weight. I have recorded as much as 30 lbs. of muscle loss due to this problem. This is not healthy weight loss, especially if there is a lot of fat gain during the same period.

Muscle Sacrificing

This is a situation where muscle is used for energy and sacrifices itself to the body for fuel purposes. It sounds odd, but it does happen. It happens if you are in a starvation situation, or when the body has an insufficient amount of calories to burn. This usually comes from eating a low caloric diet. These types of "diets" can force your body to use muscle as an alternate energy source. Unfortunately, during this period, the body often holds onto fat as an insurance policy for any future starvation! The body views starvation as a stressful situation and will hold onto remaining fat, or it may add extra fat, while sacrificing your muscle if you're not currently using it.

Client Result:

> A female client went to a well known "weight loss" clinic and lost 16 lbs. of muscle but gained six pounds of fat. This was a result of their attempted low-cal "weight loss" strategy. The 10 lbs. "loss" was a psychological boost, yet in reality, she had lost and gained the wrong kind of weight, as discovered by a body composition scan. After 12 months of training she is now in a healthy weight condition.

This experience and many others similar to it have made me realize that it is impossible to starve a fat cell!

My recommendation is:

> Do not attempt any low caloric diets, especially those which are promoting 800-1200 calories per day.

Sarcopenia

This is a natural muscle loss which usually occurs with age, but can show up as early as age 35. It usually begins to accelerate by age 60, even if you have large heavy muscles. It also can occur if there are hormonal imbalances, especially a lack of testosterone, which applies for both sexes. Lack of exercise, inadequate food intake, or a stressful lifestyle, can also contribute to the onset of sarcopenia. Men can begin to lose testosterone starting at age 45. Females can also begin losing testosterone and progesterone as early as age 42. I recommend that you start to monitor your levels beginning at these ages.

Maintaining or improving your muscle strength and weight gives you many advantages. I encourage you to have a lifelong program of resistance training which you enjoy and take pride in. Remember, you only get stronger with some form of resistance!

In the next step we will look at fat and fat weight.

Fat loss & losing
the right kind of fat

Brace yourself; the diet and weight loss industry is a billion dollar industry that really does not want you to succeed at reaching your weight control goals. It provides confusing information and protocols that offer you weight loss without telling you what *kind* of weight you will be losing even if you are successful with their plan.

Was I being a little harsh with that statement? Well, you be the judge. How many people do you know who have had not much success on these programs, or, they have 'lost weight' yet when they leave the program, they gain it all back again? You should meet all of *my* clients and people who have come to me after having that happen to them through "weight loss" programs and centers. It's staggering. Here are some of the most popular 'weight-loss' methods:

- Diet & eating plans
- Meal replacements & 'weight loss' teas
- Unproven hormonal programs
- Point system nutritional plans
- Exercise videos
- Exercise equipment
- 'Weight loss' pills, powders & drugs

All of these concepts are gearing you up for failure because they *want* your failure. No offence to anyone, and I know that sounds harsh. But if you actually 'lost weight' with them, how are they going to stay in business? After all, if everyone could achieve their goals, there would be nothing left to sell, and this is not acceptable to the big businesses who are marketing the industry currently. They have power and influence in the medical, pharmaceutical, food & beverage, nutritional, and supplement industry. If you feel you have paid enough into their pockets over the past few years, you are not alone, so please keep reading and I will share some information that *they* do not want you to know about!

If your DEXA scan shows you have achieved a healthy body fat percentage, well done, this is good news! Fat has often been given a bad rap over the years, but it is very valuable to your system. It is healthy stuff; you just don't need too much or too little of it. It is important to have just the recommended amount to sustain vital energy and hormonal functions.

If your percentage is over the recommended range, I suggest you begin a fat loss program soon, as fat tends to accumulate with age. If you need or want to lose some excess body fat it is important to know that there are four different kinds of fat in the body. Only two should be targeted for fat loss purposes, as the other two are needed for metabolic requirements, and your body will hold on to them much longer than you can imagine!

The Various Kinds of Fat

1) **White adipose tissue (WAT)** is the fat that lies just below the skin, next to, or within the muscles. Also known as *storage fat*, it is the primary target for fat loss strategies, especially those that include diet, exercise and acid/alkaline balancing.

2) **Visceral fat** surrounds and protects the internal organs. This type of fat can often build up due to negative stress and hormonal imbalances. It can be a targeted fat, yet often returns to normal levels when stress and hormonal levels are in healthier ranges.

There are two other types of fat in the body that are not targeted for fat loss. They are *brown fat* and *structural fat*. They provide a valuable service for the body and do not need to be lowered.

3) **Brown fat** was designed to keep us warm when we were babies and it still provides us with a very metabolically active tissue that helps us to keep warm when we get cold. Most of it lies across our backs and neck and acts like a blanket to cover us and keep us warm. Due to its very specific purpose, it is *not* targeted for fat loss.

4) **Structural fat** is a type of fat located around the joints, and on certain extremities, such as the hands and the bottom of the heels. It performs a valuable role in the cushioning of joints, hands and feet while protecting them from repetitive activities like walking or jogging. This is definitely *not* a targeted fat. Unfortunately, we have seen "starvation" type diets result in people having sore joints and heels due to structural fat loss.

It is my intent to assist you in maintaining the valuable fat while lowering the excess storage and visceral fat that may currently be in your body. I feel confident in saying that you will be losing *the right type of fat* by following the suggestions offered in Chapter 10.

The reasons for fat gain

In the next two chapters, I will introduce leading information for the reasons why you gain fat weight, and the strategies for assisting your body to release it.

The fat gaining and releasing mechanisms are mainly designed for white fat, which is your dominant type of storage fat. Storing fat is one of the many amazing survival and protection mechanisms which your body can call into play if it senses you are under any kind of negative stress. This mechanism is also known to take effect if it feels your body is being stressed by cold, fear, hunger, drugs, chemicals, or preservatives as well. It can store fat weight as a survival mechanism in order to "feel safer". It will also do this automatically even if you try to counter-act it by reducing your food intake or by increasing your exercise levels. The body will return to a more normal state when it senses that negative stress levels are being reduced. Only when it senses that your stress levels are down will it start an internal fat burning process. This is a two way process known as the *Body Fat Regulating System*, or BFRS. The body's primal response to "insulate" and protect you by adding *more* fat within the adipose tissues is a very tough mechanism to override. Many negative stresses in your life can trigger hormonal signals to your brain which literally say, *"I'm not safe, it's time for protection, I am in fear, I need more or better food — I need to store more fat!"* It's an incredible process. It can be taking place while you are exercising and eating correctly, while leaving you wondering why the heck your fat weight is increasing.

As it turns out, this is a chemical/hormonal process taking place *within* our bodies. It is something we cannot see or feel and it took a few years to find out what this process was, and how it worked.

This is what I have learned…

In 1994 it was discovered that a hormone called *Leptin*, was the culprit for signaling the brain to store or release fat. Leptin is also an active hormone which keeps your fat levels in *balance*. Unfortunately, if too much negative stress comes into your life, it can disrupt Leptin signals received by the hypothalamus area of the brain. The brain no longer becomes receptive to it and starts to shut down its sensitivity towards burning fat and deals with the new stress instead. When the brain no longer recognizes Leptin signals, it becomes resistant to them causing what is known as *Leptin resistance*.

Leptin resistance is one of the primary reasons we gain unwanted fat.

Leptin resistance triggers the *fat gaining mechanism* (FGM) to start its job of storing extra calories during the new period of stress. The fat storage process is called *lipogenesis*. Fat enters the cells mainly by a process called *Fatty Acid Synthase* (FAS). These enzymes are dedicated to creating fat, and are especially good at converting simple sugars and carbohydrates into storage fat. Women have more lipogenic enzymes than men and tend to put on fat weight much faster. This can also mean that they will need more time in taking off the unwanted fat pounds.

Fat cells can expand like balloons to accommodate extra energy, and up to 200 lbs. of extra fat can be stored in the human body! There are many reasons for fat gain and it is a bit of a sleuthing role on your part to discover which one (or more) is triggering *your* fat gaining mechanism. Think of what may be happening to your life right now to make you feel stressed. It may answer questions as to why you are having problems with fat weight gain.

Here are some of the most common scenarios:

1) **Negative or chronic stress and fear**. This often triggers an increase in cortisol levels (the fight or flight response hormone) which has a negative effect on the fat burning process. Chronically elevated levels of cortisol can maintain fat gains and have a negative impact on your overall health.

2) **Insulin resistance**. This is a situation that can be brought on by eating too many simple sugars and foods which convert easily to glucose, a type of sugar that can be transported into the cells for energy. Insulin acts as a carrier of glucose and is needed to 'open doors' of cellular walls. Too much glucose is toxic to cells and they respond by shutting down insulin receptor sites on these walls. When this happens glucose builds up in the blood, causing *high blood glucose*, and high circulating blood insulin levels, or *hyperinsulinemia*. Both can increase fat gain. Foods which contain these simple sugars are soft drinks, candy, baked goods, pasta, rice and potatoes.

3)   **Acidosis.** The body recognizes acid as a toxic substance and will store it in fat cells as a natural detoxifying method within the body. The more acidic you become the more fat you will tend to store.

5)   **Sluggish or toxic liver**. The liver metabolizes fat and cannot process it efficiently if it is clogged or full of waste.

6)   **Hormonal Imbalances**. Proper functioning of the *endocrine system* (pineal, hypothalamus, pituitary, thyroid and adrenal glands) is essential for keeping fat in healthy levels. For example, an under active thyroid (*hypothyroidism*) can slow down your metabolism and cause fat gains.

7)   **Overeating**. This is very common, especially if you like all you can eat sushi bars! It includes all types of food including fat, protein and carbohydrates. Almost all food eaten can be converted to fat and stored in fat cells, making any food potentially "fattening" if eaten in excess. The DEXA scan will give you an approximate daily caloric intake which suits your current situation. Quite often, extra calories means extra fat weight, as the body stores extra food for its "backup" system.

8)   **Under eating**. Starvation and starvation type diets (low-caloric) initially seem like a good idea, but you cannot starve a fat cell! The body will respond to low caloric intake

in exactly the opposite way that you might have intended or thought. It will slow down and use fewer calories, plus it will store more calories instead in the form of fat to protect itself for the reduced food intake it is experiencing.

Client example:

I measured a woman before and after a low caloric diet. After a seven month period, she lost 18 lbs. of muscle and gained six pounds of fat! The initial happiness of a 12 lbs. 'weight loss' was quickly lost when she discovered she had gained and lost the wrong kind of weight. Every time you try to "diet" you can actually end up gaining fat. The average fat gain is 11 lbs.!

9)   **Lack of exercise**. Exercise avoidance can slow down your results considerably for overall fat loss, as it is vital for burning excess blood sugars and for revving up your metabolism that can assist in fat loss.

10)   **Pineal or Hypothalamus stress** due to toxic overload. This one is important! Not just for fat loss but for overall health! Research has shown that a damaged or stressed pineal or hypothalamus gland will increase fat weight substantially, often due to neurotoxin stress. Substances and toxins that need to be avoided or given up completely include the following:

- Food additives and preservatives (especially excitotoxins like MSG and aspartame)
- Artificial flavorings, dyes and emulsifiers
- Artificial sweeteners such as high fructose corn syrup, saccharin, aspartame (brand names are *NutraSweet, Equal & Spoonful*), sucralose, acesulfame, & neotame
- Heavy metal ingestion; this includes avoiding high mercury levels in some fish species (tuna) and avoiding vaccinations as they contain *thimersol*, a mercury based preservative (tough one to do…)
- Food that has been sprayed with pesticides and herbicides
- Soft drinks; they contain artificial sweeteners and may contain subtle fluoride toxins
- Fluoridated water
- Smoking or second hand smoke
- Genetically modified foods (GMO)

It is important to realize that your body was designed to insulate and protect you with the fat gaining mechanism. It served us well in ancient times as it was often the "survival of the fattest" which kept the human race going. In today's world we can still trigger those ancient safeguards.

Please remember: gaining fat weight or getting fatter is not a disease or a medical

condition, it is just one of your body's many
survival and protection mechanisms.

Early detection and recognition of stressors that
cause excess fat gain can assist you in reaching
personal fat loss goals. Be aware of what triggers
your fat gaining mechanism into action. There are
many strategies for losing fat effectively and
naturally – and we'll go over those in the next
chapter!

How to lose unwanted fat

As mentioned in the last chapter, the body will often return to a healthy fat weight percentage once stressful emotional, nutritional and lifestyle situations are alleviated. The overall concept is to avoid stimulating the FGM while stimulating the abilities of the *fat releasing mechanism* (FRM). This fat releasing process is called *lipolysis*. There are enzymes which help the release of fat from cells called *lipolytic enzymes*. Females have less of these enzymes than males, which can often make fat loss harder for them.

If you need or want to lose some excess body fat, here are the top ten natural, drug free, strategies that have proven to be successful for the past ten years. These strategies become even more effective as we grow older.

Finally, the Top 10 Strategies

1) **Discover and *reduce* the negative stressors in your life**. As mentioned before, everyone responds to stress in a different way. Find out which stressors affect you in a negative way. If you think about a problem more than five times a day, this can be a identified as a negative stress in your life. Negative stress may come from a variety of situations such as physical pain, emotional trauma, mental fatigue, food additives, and/or environmental pollutants.

   Client Example:

   Sherri, one of my favorite clients, had a hard time releasing her husband, who was unfortunately giving her chronic stress. After their separation she lost 18 lbs. of fat in seven months.

2) **Avoid Leptin resistance**. Eating a low carbohydrate and low sugar diet can assist in keeping Leptin in balance. Also avoid all food additives, preservatives, chemicals, artificial flavors, environmental pollutants, solvents and chemical cleaners. They all can prompt negative stress in the body.   Keeping a Leptin balance in your body is vital for fat loss, as it gives the brain messages which say, "*It's safe, let's release the stored fat*".

3) **Avoid Insulin Resistance**. Similar to Leptin resistance, insulin resistance can become a chronic stress if you ingest a high sugar/grain

diet. Avoid all sugars and food that converts easily to sugar such as soft drinks and bread. Reduce consumption of *high glycemic foods* such as grains, sweetbreads, cookies, cakes, rice, and cooked potatoes. Avoid all artificial sweeteners such as Splenda, NutraSweet, aspartame, saccharine and acesulfame. Avoid products that contain high sucrose, fructose, maltose and dextrose.

Note:

Insulin resistance used to be called diabetes or *diabetes mellitus*, which translates into "sweet urine flowing through body". This describes a symptom, and in fact for many years it was known as "sweet urine disease". Diabetes is not a disease, it is only a made up name that describes a symptom of a much deeper root issue which is usually elevated blood sugar (EBS,) or insulin resistance. I recommend avoiding all drugs for managing blood glucose (sugar) levels. They can often cause the condition to worsen.   I also recommend having your blood glucose levels checked on a regular basis and make an intention to keep them in healthy ranges.

Recommended Fasting Glucose Levels are between 2.5 - 6.5 mmol/L.

4)   **Achieve and maintain high alkaline levels**. In an ideal world your body prefers to be in a slightly alkaline as most biochemical and hormonal exchanges work better in this state. For example:

Ideal blood pH is **7.365 - 7.4**. Maintaining a diet that is two thirds alkaline foods and one third acids will contribute to a better alkaline state.

Other tips include:

1. Consume filtered natural water that has a pH of 7.5 or higher. Avoid fluoridated water and all substances that contain fluoride, including fluoride mouthwashes and toothpaste. It is a toxin that can play havoc with the brain, thyroid and the bones.
2. Avoiding long strenuous workouts as this can often generate more acid in your body.
3. Practicing diaphragmatic breathing while exercising. This helps to lower the amount of *carbonic acid* which is produced in your system.
4. Avoid all drugs, preservatives, additives, sugar, and negative stress. These all contribute to a more acidic body as well.
5. Get a restful sleep at night, eat natural organic food when possible. Go outside and breathe deeply to receive more oxygen. All of these contribute to a more alkaline state.
6. Check your pH levels on a regular basis.
7. **Practice *metabolic* eating.**

Metabolic eating greatly helps you avoid the starvation response, assists your thyroid in functioning, keeps you in balance, and helps you burn fat effectively. This is a good life long approach for eating, and is not just a short term diet or food replacement program. Here are key points to metabolic eating:

1.   Eat a large protein and "good" fat breakfast. An example would be a three egg vegetable omelet. Add Essential fatty acids (EFA's) such as fish oil or Omega 3 *good* oils with the meal.

2.   Attempt to eat 3 meals per day, each one being the size of your wrist and fist. Attempt to have 2-3 snacks every day, the size of three fingers. This helps digestion, assimilation, elimination, and thyroid functions.

3.   Attempt a food program which consists of 70 - 80% alkaline foods per day. This helps to keep you in a healthy alkaline state and maintains a high level of natural digestive enzymes within your system. Have as much raw food as you can handle.

4.   Avoid simple sugars and foods which convert to sugar easily such as soft drinks, rice, grains and baked goods.

5.   Avoid overeating. Try the *80% Rule*. Eat until you are 80% full, and then stop. Do not eat until you are full as it prompts the storage of excess calories as fat. This is a major problem which may need some serious attention!

6.   Avoid under eating. Feed your body well! You want to eat good natural whole food all day, each day, to prevent the

starvation response (FGM), while giving the body what it needs.

7. Avoid a large meal or eating after 7:30pm. The body starts to slow down its metabolism rate after this time and does not process food well.

8. Hydrate as often as possible with to aid in the digestive and elimination process.

9. If you want or need sweeteners, try *Stevia* (a natural herb), organic unpasteurized honey or maple syrup.

10. Enjoy your food! Make meals colorful, have them in pleasurable surroundings, and enjoy them with family and friends. As they say "let food be your medicine".

5) **Practice a regular *detoxification* program, especially one for the liver.** One of the liver's many functions are to break down fats. A congested liver full of toxins cannot breakdown fats effectively and extra fat storage is a common result. Extra toxins can be stored in fat cells, and we have seen as much as 8 lbs. of fat and toxin loss as a result of specific detoxifying programs.

Note:

Toxic weight loss is the only other weight besides fat that is considered to be a healthy loss.

We have recorded a lot of toxic weight loss alone due to what is known as "compacted" fecal matter in the colon, and our colonic therapist says that up to 10 lbs. of toxic loss is not uncommon! Here are some common detoxification programs:

- Ionic foot- spa detoxification
- Herbal detox formulas
- Far infrared saunas
- Colonic irrigation therapy

Client Result:

Barry came to me after suffering a 6 month long full body infected rash from the toxic effects of an H1N1 vaccination. He was very self conscious and had spent over $3000 on medications from physicians. I explained that it could be a mercury or aluminum problem and that the detoxification foot - spa system that I have at my clinic might help the condition (it has the ability to remove a lot of heavy metals from the body). After only five sessions the rash was 90% gone and Barry, feeling much more confident, was able to begin his health program and lose eight pounds of fat.

6) **Maintain a *regular* fitness and activity program**. Absolutely essential for a healthy life, exercise is great for burning off extra blood sugars and helping lower your stored fat. Exercise three to four times per week for optimal benefits. Exercise needs to be done correctly though, in order to receive its many benefits. I recommend a new Anabolic Cross training system that has been proven to be very successful for many people. I will take

extra time out to show what it is, how to do it, and explain its benefits.

First of all, *anabolic* means to "build up", which is what this workout can do for your fitness and health parameters. It is also intended to help maintain or build up your bone and muscle content while decreasing your fat percentage.

Quite often an exercise program can be too stressful on the body, and as a result, it begins to "break down" from the exercises. This is known as a *catabolic* situation. This is not what you want to happen, and this is why I designed a great simple workout that builds up your body and your current fitness levels. The overall intent of the workout is to provide you with:

- A comprehensive workout that keeps you in your *Target Heart Rate Zone* for 40 - 60 minutes
- Variety and diversity to prevent repetitive injuries, or boredom
- Easy to follow exercises which can be done outside or in the gym
- A program based on your needs and exercises that you prefer
- A program that offers you faster results with less time commitments
- A program that is easy to follow and thus easier to do more often

This basic program combines three to four cardio workouts with a good amount of resistance exercise that are performed in a continuous manner with little or no rest breaks. Note: bring along a resistance band if you are exercising outdoors.

Step 1) *Warm-up and Cardio*

Begin with any cardio exercise (treadmill, bike, walking etc.). Spend the first three minutes warming up and bring your heart rate to 65% of your maximum Heart Rate Target Zone (HRTZ). Then raise the heart rate over the next 5 - 8 minutes to your 65% to 80% HRTZ. Stop and walk for 10-15 seconds.

Step 2) *Resistance Session*

Find a spot to perform 10 - 15 reverse lunges. Next, find a spot where you can do 10 - 15 push-ups (on your knees or on an angle is good to start). Find soft ground or a mat and finish with 20 sit-ups.

Step 3) *Cardio*

Continue your walk-jog if you are outside, or find a cardio machine if you are in the gym, and move your heart rate back into your HRTZ for 5 minutes.

Step 4) *Resistance Session*

If you are outside, use resistance bands for 10 - 15 repetitions of bicep curls, triceps press down, and shoulder presses. If you are indoors, use machines or free weights to perform these three exercises (pick light to medium weights).

Step 5) *Back to Cardio*

Continue with the same cardio (5 minutes) or move on to a different one for variety. If you are outside, the oxygen is really coming into your system by now, especially if DL breathing is becoming more comfortable to use.

Step 6) *Back to Resistance*

Perform 10 - 15 lateral pull-downs, 20 side sit-ups, and finish with 10 - 15 calve raises.

Step 7) *Cardio Again!*

Keep going for another 5 minutes and during the last 30 seconds, elevate your heart rate to 85% of your maximum HRTZ. Attempt to slowly integrate this 30 second "push" at the end of each cardio session for extra fat burning.

Step 8) *Last - Resistance!*

This is the last one, so it's your choice to repeat any three exercises you prefer or enjoy! Finish with a stretching session to slowly bring your heart rate down to fewer than 90 beats per minute. Talk a deep breathe, you're done!

This workout is one of my personal favorites. I especially enjoy hiking and jogging with my resistance bands in the various parks of North Vancouver.

Back to our Top 10 List

9) **Achieve and maintain healthy *Triglyceride* levels** (can be tested via a blood test). Optimal levels indicate you are *burning* fat which is a good situation. Elevated levels indicate that your body is releasing fat into the bloodstream. These levels mean that fat is being stored and sugar is being used for energy instead. This is not a good scenario. It turns you into a *sugar burner* rather than a fat burner. It can also alter your food cravings and tend to make you want to eat more foods full of sugar to satisfy this process. Since sugar energy becomes the primary energy source, it can override the fat burning process.

    Recommended ranges for triglycerides are 0.45 – 2.29mmol/L

    It is better to become a fat burner rather than a sugar burner. To assist this, you can increase your consumption of essential fatty acids, especially Omega 3 oils. It sounds counter productive, but increasing the "good fats" in your diet actually increases your ability to burn stored fat. Examples of good fats include fish oils, krill oil, olive oil, avocado oil, macadamia oil and virgin coconut oil.

10) **Maintain healthy hormonal levels**. This includes achieving and maintaining healthy levels for the thyroid, adrenals, parathyroid and reproductive glands. For females it means maintaining balanced levels of estrogen, progesterone, testosterone, DHEA and HGH. For males this also means maintaining good levels of testosterone, human growth hormone (HGH) and DHEA. Having high levels of HGH is helpful in achieving a *Healthy Weight* as it enhances the burning of fat, keeps your muscle metabolism strong and it aids in the building of strong bones as well. Many people over the age of 40 can experience a drop in their HGH levels. When we were younger our levels could have been as high as 600ug, but as we age, we often need hormonal help!

HGH aids our cells by helping them function correctly. Fat cells are one of the target cells of HGH. It helps to break down triglycerides and also suppress their ability to accumulate circulating blood fats. This also helps *carbohydrate metabolism*, and assists in maintaining healthy blood sugar levels. HGH is truly a master hormone and assists the body in many positive ways. It can be measured and monitored by using an indicator test called the insulin growth factor (IGF-1). There are no current recommended levels for HGH, but the higher your levels are, the better it is for long term health benefits.

There are natural supplements available that can increase HGH levels. They include:

- Colostrum
- L-argine
- L-lysine
- L-glutamine
- Phosphatidylcholine

Supplements are often sold in health food stores as 'HGH releasers' as it can enhance the release of HGH from the brain. I have recorded increases from these supplements in as little as six months. Note, contact an experienced health professional for assistance in this area.

We Hope You Enjoyed That Very Long List

A word about "weight loss" supplements and "diet pills" is next. There are many products and drugs that are marketed as weight loss tools. These products often target *fat loss, although most do not suggest what kind of "weight" they are targeting.* Some can unfortunately cause metabolic damage in the process. This means that they often cause the body to lose water, muscle or bone in the so called "weight loss" process, and they often have very negative side effects. They are:

- **Thermogenic promoters**. They attempt to "rev up" the metabolism, usually with some kind of stimulant in hopes of "burning more calories" (i.e. *Cylaris, Hydroxycut & Lipofuse).*

- **Appetite suppressants** (satiety enhancers). The most common is an African herb called Hoodia. Bush tribesmen are said to eat it to help them suppress their appetites in order to last days without food (i.e. *Trimspa* and *Phentermine*). Some diet pills work to make you feel full all the time (such as *Sibutramine*)!

- **Hormone reducers**. Cortisol is raised when the body is under stress, and marketers have promoted the concept that cortisol increases "belly fat". Logic then says, "Let's market a product that lowers cortisol". It sounds good but the body does not like any of its natural functions to be tampered with for very long (i.e. *Relacore*).

- **Hormone altering**. The most recent treatment is once a week injections with human chorionic gonadotrohin, (HCG) coupled with a low protein, and low caloric diet. HCG is intended to stimulate the hypothalamus to release stored fat for the fetus in pregnant females. This treatment was tried 50 years ago, and like today, often produces muscle loss as its main "weight loss" due to the reduced caloric intake. Like most "diets" it deprives you of nutrients, produces light headiness, low energy, short term fat loss, and never really allows your body to rely on its natural abilities to help you achieve a healthy weight. It can be very expensive, has negative side effects, and no real long term solutions.

- **Insulin resistance and glucose lowering pills.** These products attempt to aid the body in lowering the amount of circulating blood glucose (i.e. *Glucofast*).

- **Fat blockers**. They attempt to block fat absorption often with nasty side effects (i.e. *Xenical/Orlistat, Chitosan & Alli*).

- **Carbohydrate blockers**. They attempt to block carbohydrate absorption and thus hope to block more glucose from entering the fat cells (i.e. *C-Block & 5 - HTP*).

- **Detoxification supplements**. These pills attempt to help clean the body of built up toxins, which is not a bad idea, just check labels (i.e. *Ororo - Detox, Cleansonix*).

All of these "weight loss" drugs or supplements contain ingredients that may have some benefit, but most are promoting an artificial or short term way to lose "weight" or fat. Since they do not suggest or name the type of weight or the type of fat they are targeting, it is a buyer-beware scenario. They often block natural functions of the body by tricking the body into doing something that is not natural or healthy in the long run. I have not seen or heard of any long term changes made with any one supplement or drug.

Beware the Drugs & Pills

"Weight loss" on drugs will always plateau, as you are providing another artificial way to hold back the BFRS. This system will eventually find a way around the drugs but they often leave the body in a damaged way. Many can do permanent damage to your system and therefore, I recommend using only the top 10 natural methods to remedy fat loss. All of these methods contribute to a healthy lifestyle and can help you to keep off the excess fat weight for life. Please be aware of any *weight loss* product or program. Their promotions are usually for the short term, with little or no regard for your long term health. They will often offer fast results with no pain, or promise things like "eat all that you want without exercising". More often than not, the weight that you lose is muscle or water, which is *not* the type of weight you may need or want to lose. Don't be fooled by the hype of *weight loss*, you need to know *what* kind of weight you are losing or gaining on any diet or weight control program!

The people who we see lose the most fat, and keep it off for the long term, do so by making complete lifestyle changes.

If something happens and you slip off your regular lifestyle patterns and gain back extra fat weight, remember the Top 10 Tips list! They act as great guides for fat loss and can be used at anytime in your quest for a healthier lifestyle.

Thinking differently about your weight

Here is the most important concept to grasp in order to shift your thinking about weight:

> When you stand on the scale the number you see only measures the total amount of *all* your weights, and is actually *not* an indicator of what you should or shouldn't weigh, or what a healthy weight is for you.

This is also true for any other weight measuring or monitoring program, especially those using height/weight charts. These measuring systems in the past attempted to describe what a healthy weight was, yet failed to take into consideration that the body can shift its active weights many times during the course of a life time.

My new model provides accurate and current information for determining which of your active weights need to be adjusted to meet your needs. Body composition assessments, coupled with information on natural ways to achieve a healthy weight, are a practical solution for all of your goals.

Here again is the new definition for a *healthy weight*:

> *A healthy weight is achieved when all of your active weights are within recommended levels.*

Your thoughts on weight may be beginning to shift, and in order for them to really change on this subject, I would like you to throw away the bathroom scale, or put it in storage for the next nine months! If you have done this and have taken a DEXA scan, you are well on your way to developing a positive lifelong approach to your weight control.

I feel that you deserve a body that is full of energy, a mind capable of great vision and a spirit that is unafraid to dream big dreams.

This is the true and real state of health that is available to you and your family when you are dedicated to promoting the basic natural processes of your life. If you follow the suggestions that have been provided in this book, there is a good possibility that your body will return to a more natural state, and be in recommended body composition ranges in as little as nine months.

Remember, being within these ranges is the overall goal, and it can also help you to begin a more natural, healthy, and balanced life. When you wake up tomorrow, plan to do as many things as possible that will create a healthier you. Plan to begin your intents, goals and action steps so that they can truly benefit you for the rest of your life.

I wish you all the best in your pursuit of a healthier lifestyle.

Thank you for reading my first book.

In Health,
Allan Lawry

If you have any questions about body weight, *The Healthy Weight® Program*, or achieving a *Healthy Weight*, please contact Allan Lawry at his website, allanlawry.com, or send him an email at info@allanlawry.com today.

Thank you.

Signup to his mailing list to become the first to be notified about his next up and coming book:

Osteoporosis – Disease or Healer?

Nobody Is Overweight

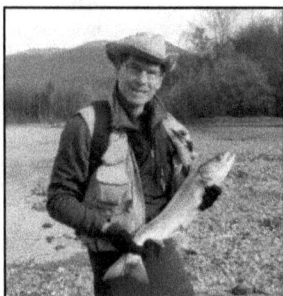

Fitness and Lifestyle Coach, Allan Lawry, has designed a revolutionary weight control method called the Healthy Weight® Program. It is rapidly becoming the program of choice for those wanting the most current, accurate and proven methods for long-term natural results.

Based on the science of body composition scans and leading strategies for adjusting fat, muscle and bone into recommended levels, Allan's concepts are unique and based on 25 years of knowledge and results. They are now available to you. His new model for weight control is gaining support across Canada due to its practical and scientific approach.

Discover why you are not overweight, and join the new way to manage your weight for life! More information on joining is located on the back of this page.

www.ingramcontent.com/pod-product-compliance
Lightning Source LLC
Chambersburg PA
CBHW072207270326
41930CB00011B/2561